I0844993

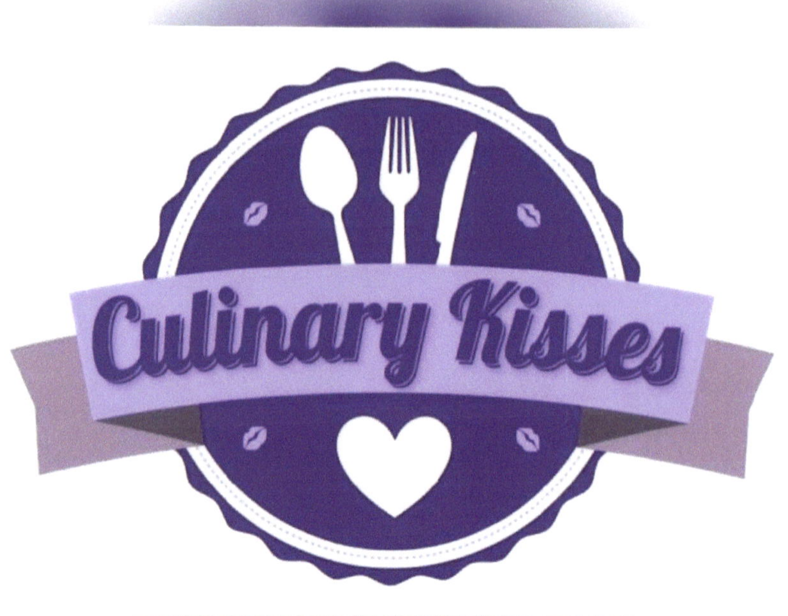

Chef Angela-Michelle

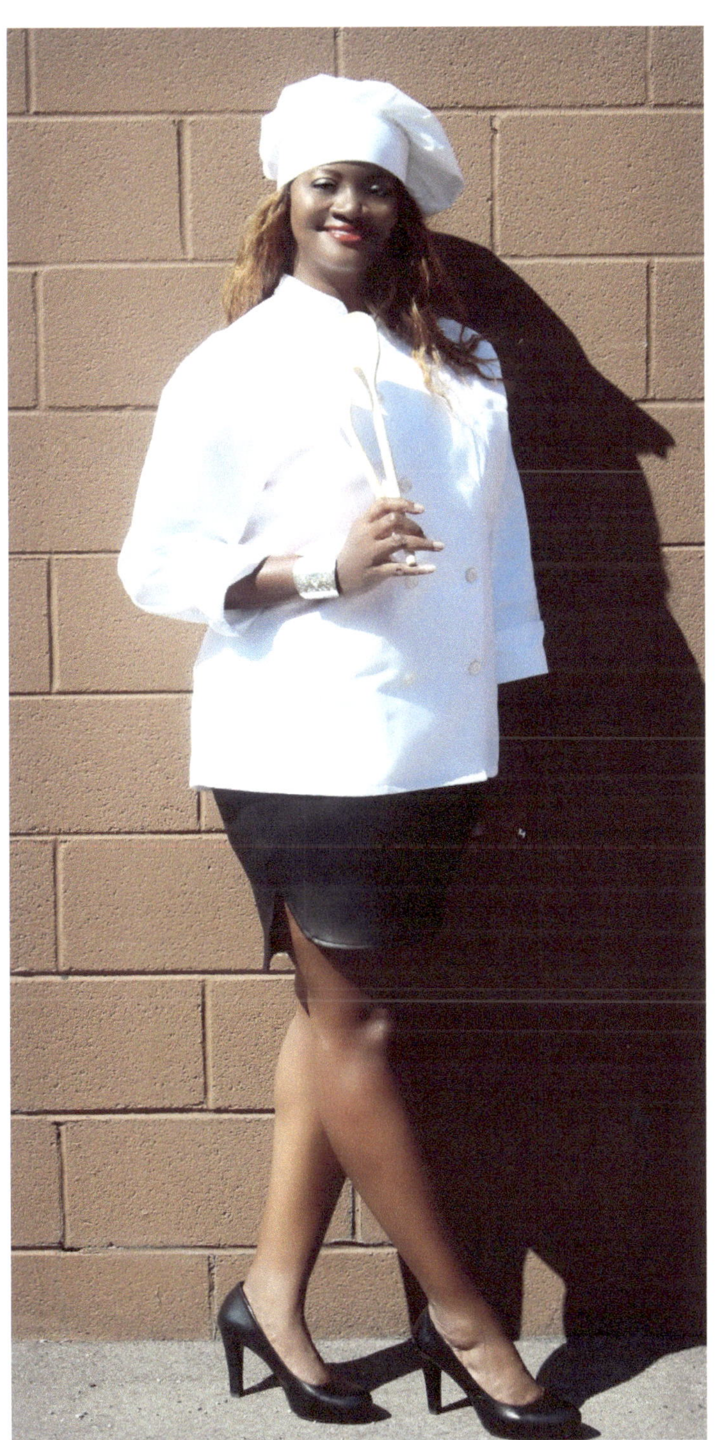

The Culinary Kisses

5 - D A Y   D E T O X
A   M A D E   E A S Y
M E A L - P L A N

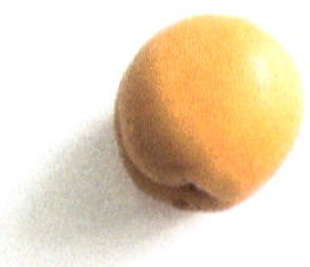

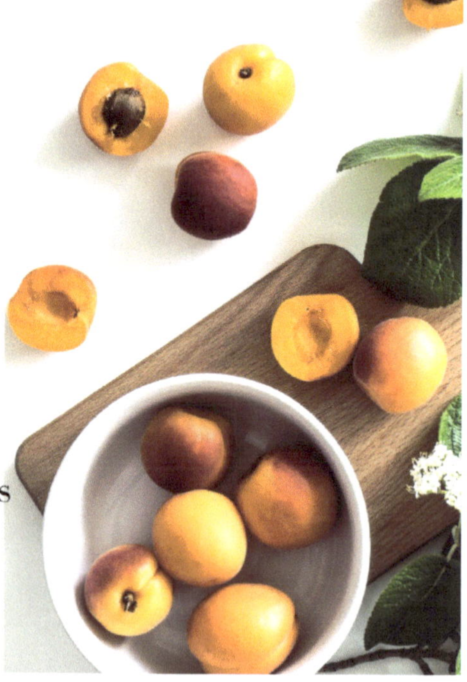

www.CulinaryKisses.com

INTRODUCTION

The 5-Day Detox Program is a temporary adjustment to your diet with the purpose of riding your body of toxins and other unhealthy substances. Almost anyone can use this program to cleanse their body. It's easy, effective, and doesn't require any outlandish ingredients. There may be some food options listed below that you've never heard of or tasted before, but there are also plenty of familiar food options listed. All of these options should be available to purchase from your local grocery store. As a matter of fact, you may already have a number of them in your pantry or refrigerator.

How often you detox is up to you. It's a personal decision. The great thing about this program is it can be used anytime. As always, consult with your physician before changing your diet.

Now here are some details, tips, and guidelines to help you on your detox journey …

DETAILS

Breakfast - smoothie with non-dairy milk, green leafy vegetable, fruit, seeds, vegetable protein powder, etc.

Snack - fruit, nuts, seeds, plain air-popped popcorn, non-dairy yogurt, granola

Lunch - vegetables, beans, grains, fruit

Dessert - fresh fruit, fruit sorbet, fruit and chia seed pudding

Snack - fruit, nuts, seeds, plain air-popped popcorn, non-dairy yogurt, granola

Dinner - large salad with homemade salad dressing

THE CULINARY KISSES 5-DAY DETOX: A MADE-EASY MEAL PLAN

<u>GUIDELINES</u>

1. No dairy, gluten, meat, processed food, fast food, junk food, sodas, flavored water, or fried food

2. Reduce or eliminate sodium, sugar, and all food from any kind of container or package

3. Drink more water, eat more fruit and vegetables, and increase physical activity

4. Eat regularly, like every 3-4 hours, in small portion sizes

5. Drink only plain water and plain tea or tea with a very little raw honey

6. Use organic produce, if possible

7. Eat healthy fats only (i.e. avocado, walnuts, coconut, etc)

<u>TIPS</u>

1. Shop the outside perimeter of the grocery store only. To save on money, buy the fresh produce that's on sale.

2. Buy produce from a local Farmer's Market.

3. Remove tempters ... all tempting foods that fall outside of the guidelines must go.

5. Read labels to make sure you're following the guidelines.

6. Prepare your meals and snacks ahead of time.

7. Dance while watching your favorite half hour TV show (and rest during commercials) to get some cardio in.

MEAL PLAN

This is a sample of the 5-DAY DETOX Program. Feel free to use it as a guide for your detox, or to use it as a template to create your our meal plan. Just remember to follow the detox guidelines and you can't go wrong.

5-Day Detox Meal Plan

	BREAKFAST	LUNCH	SNACKS	DINNER
MONDAY	Fruit and Greens Smoothie	Grain + Vegetable + Bean	Herbal Tea and Raw Almonds	Large Salad with Homemade Dressing
TUESDAY	Non-Dairy Yogurt with Fresh Fruit and Homemade Granola	Grain + Vegetable + Root + Other	Spa Water with Raw Nuts	Large Salad with Homemade Dressing
WEDNESDAY	Fruit and Greens Smoothie	Grain + Vegetable + Bean	Coconut Water with Raw Nuts	Large Salad with Homemade Dressingt
THURSDSAY	Non-Dairy Yogurt with Fresh Fruit and Homemade Granola	Grain + Vegetable + Root + Other	Herbal Tea and Raw Almonds	Large Salad with Homemade Dressing
FRIDAY	Fruit and Greens Smoothie	Grain + Vegetable + Bean	Spa Water with Raw Nuts	Large Salad with Homemade Dressing
SATURDAY	MAKE	A	GOOD	DECISION
SUNDAY	EAT	THE	RAINBOW	!!!

DETOX SMOOTHIES

Strawberry Smoothie Delight

Ingredients:

1/4 cup organic Tuscan kale
1/4 cup organic baby spinach
2 tbsp. organic old fashioned oats
1/2 tsp organic Ceylon cinnamon
1 cup organic frozen strawberries
1/2 tbsp. organic raw blue agave
1 1/2 cups organic almond milk

Instructions:

1. Blend
2. Drink
3. Enjoy

Notes:

You can alter this recipe to make it your own. Feel free to add or replace ingredients, while keeping the detox guidelines in mind.

My Quote of the Day ... "If you're going to be, you might as well be great!"

"Strawberry Smoothie Delight"

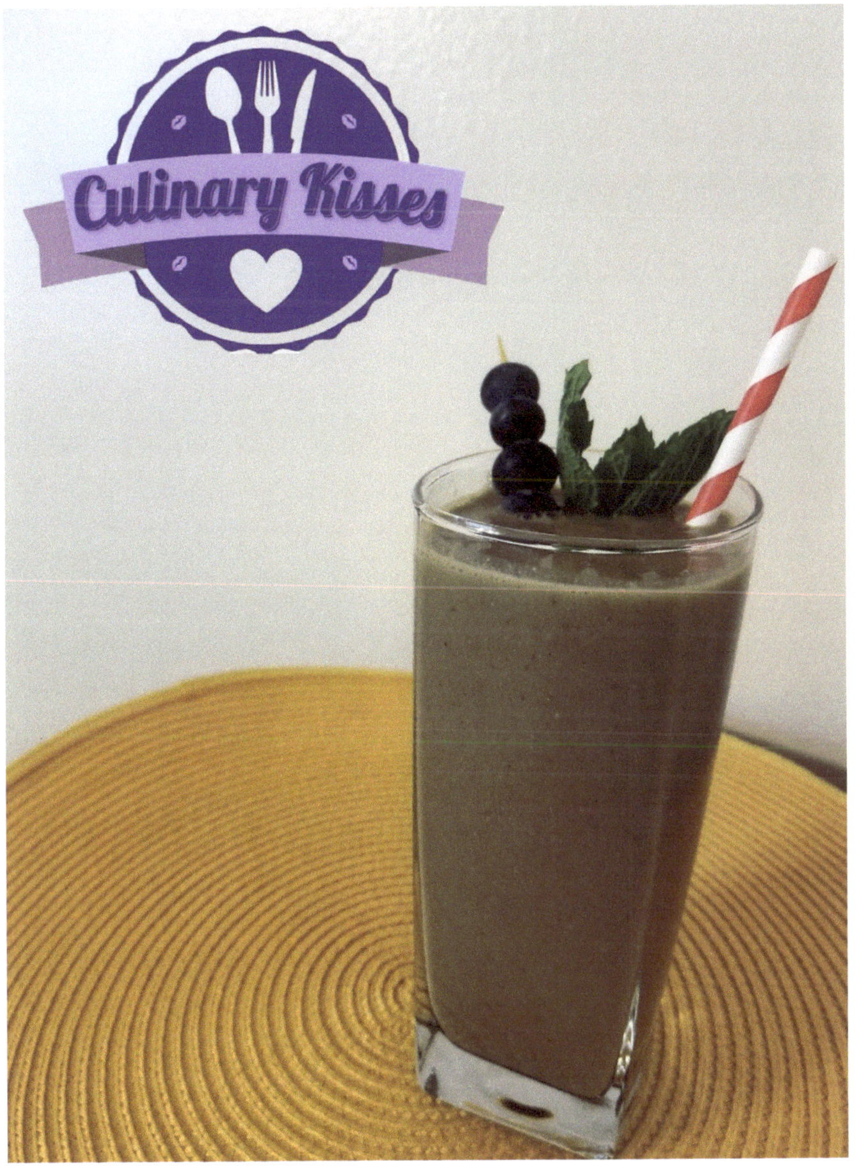

Mighty Mango Smoothie

Ingredients:

A pinch organic Tuscan kale
1/2 cup organic baby spinach
2 organic pitted dates
A drop of vanilla bean paste or vanilla extract
1/4 tsp organic ground nutmeg
1 cup organic frozen mango
1 1/2 cups organic almond milk

Instructions:

1. Blend
2. Drink
3. Enjoy

Notes:

Don't be thrown off by the color. Even though the smoothie is green (because of the tender, sweet baby spinach), it has a delightful taste that's pleasing to the palette.

My Quote of the Day ... "Fear limits your blessings and stops your potential ... So go forward & live a fearless life!"

THE CULINARY KISSES 5-DAY DETOX: A MADE-EASY MEAL PLAN

"Mighty Mango Smoothie"

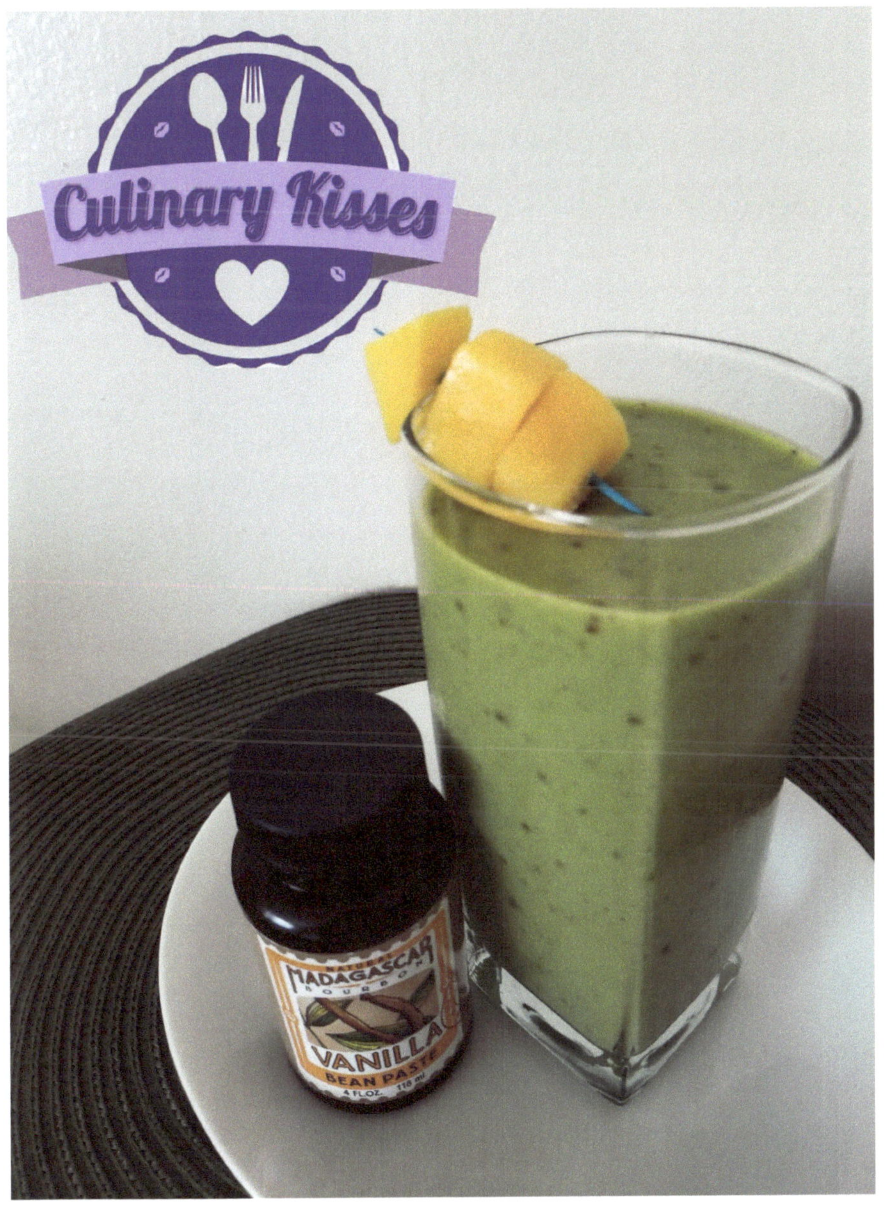

Boomtastic Blueberry Smoothie

Ingredients:

1/2 cup organic Tuscan kale
1 cup frozen blueberries
1 tbsp. organic raw pumpkin seeds
1 1/2 tbsp. organic old fashioned oats
1 tbsp. organic raw blue agave
1 1/2 cups organic almond milk

Instructions:

1. Blend
2. Drink
3. Enjoy

Notes:
This smoothie gives you a boost in antioxidants that can help protect cells from damage caused by free radicals. So with that being said, I think the old saying should be changed to "a smoothie a day keeps the doctor away."

My Quote of the Day … "Take your wildest dreams, multiple them by 100, and realize you deserve all of that and so much more."

"Boomtastic Blueberry Smoothie"

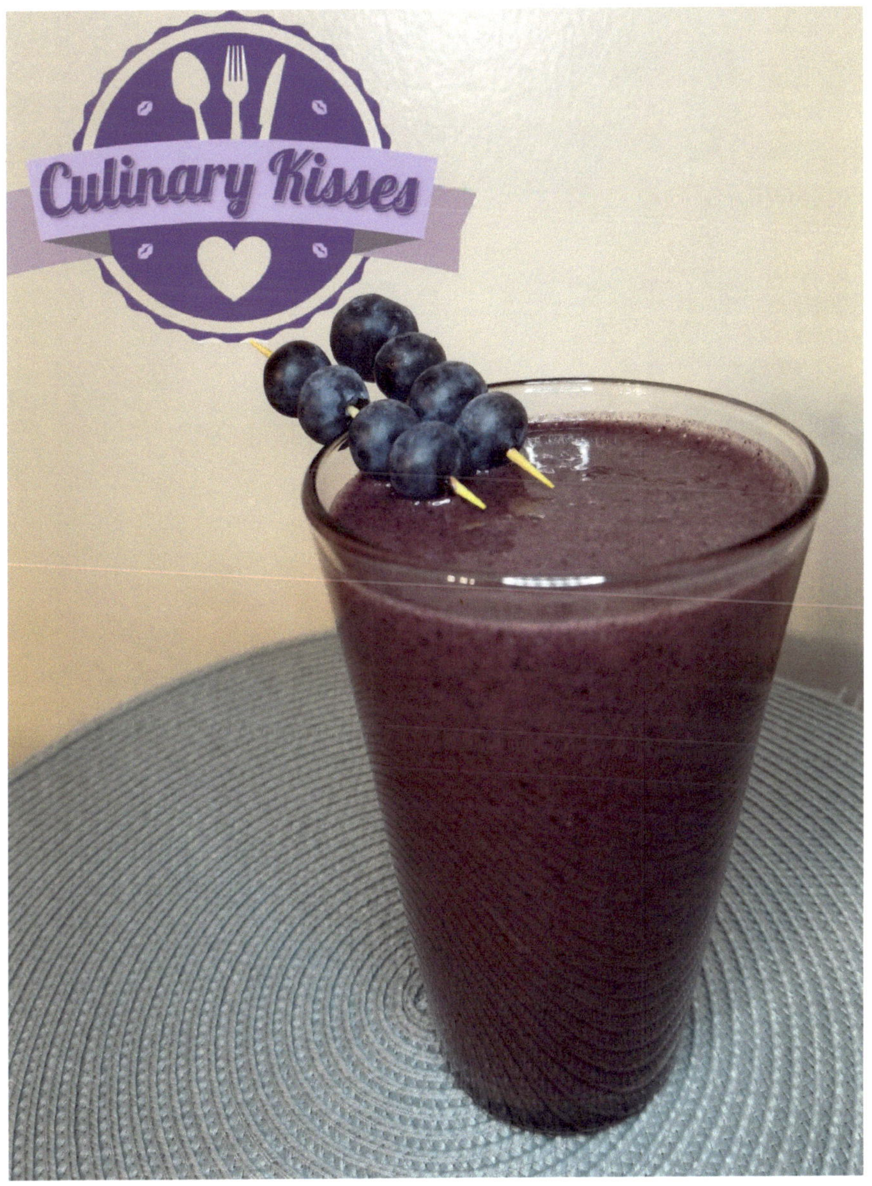

Pina Colada Smoothie

Ingredients:

1 cup organic baby spinach
1 cup organic frozen pineapple chunks
1 tbsp. organic raw blue agave
1/4 cup organic shaved coconut
1/2 tsp organic ground allspice
1 tsp organic vanilla bean paste or 1/2 tsp vanilla extract
1/4 cup organic raw walnut pieces
1 1/2 cup organic almond milk

Instructions:

1. Blend
2. Drink
3. Enjoy

Notes:
Even though this version of a Pina Colada doesn't have any alcohol, it still has a taste that is undeniable.

My Quote of the Day ... "The light inside of you is beautiful and uniquely yours, so protect and treasure it, no matter what!"

"Pina Colada Smoothie"

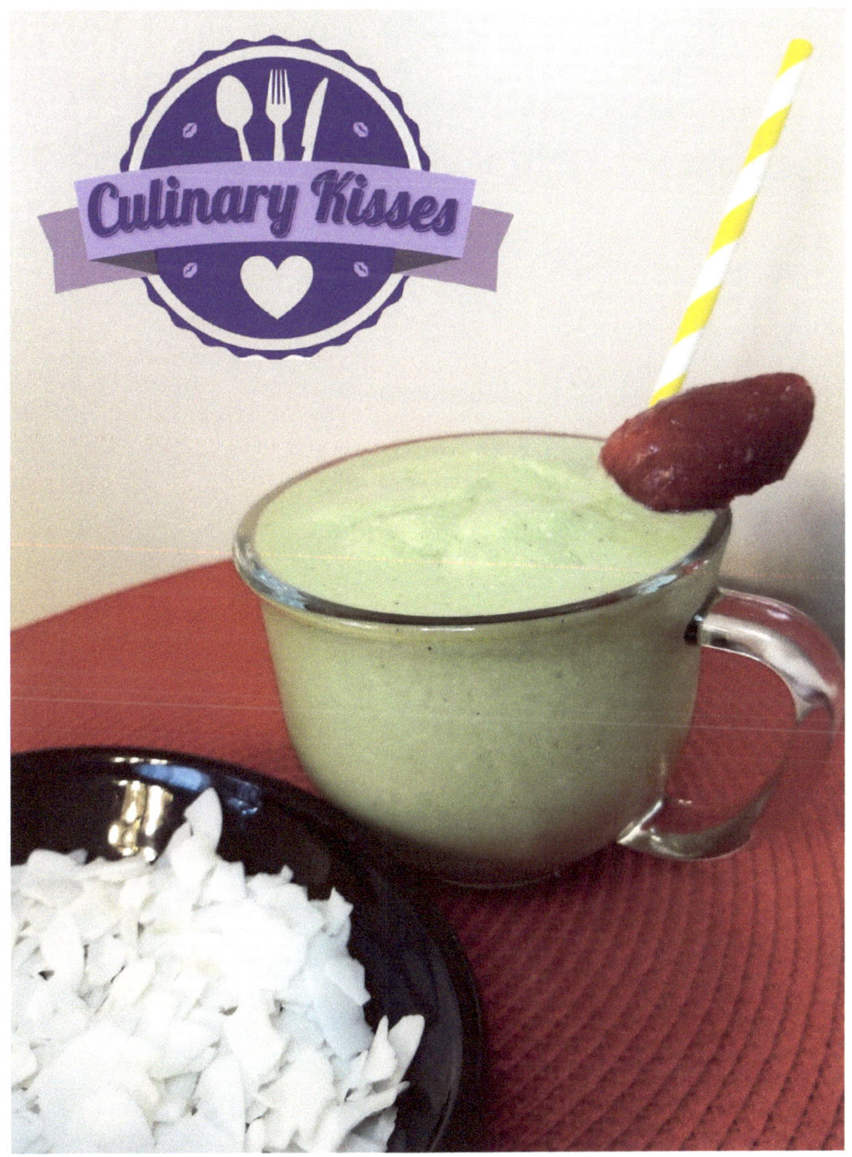

Tropical Blast Smoothie

Ingredients:

1/4 cup organic Tuscan kale
1/4 cup organic baby spinach
1/4 cup frozen pineapple chunks
3-4 frozen strawberries
1/4 cup frozen mango chunks
1 1/2 tbsp. organic old fashioned oats
1 tbsp. organic raw blue agave
1/4 cup organic raw walnut pieces
A dash of ground cinnamon
1 1/2 cup organic almond milk

Instructions:

1. Blend
2. Drink
3. Enjoy

Notes:

You can't go wrong with pineapples, strawberries, and mangoes. No
further explanation required. (LOL)

My Quote for the Day ... "You are who you say you are, so only
speak greatness (even if you don't feel like it)!"

"Tropical Blast Smoothie"

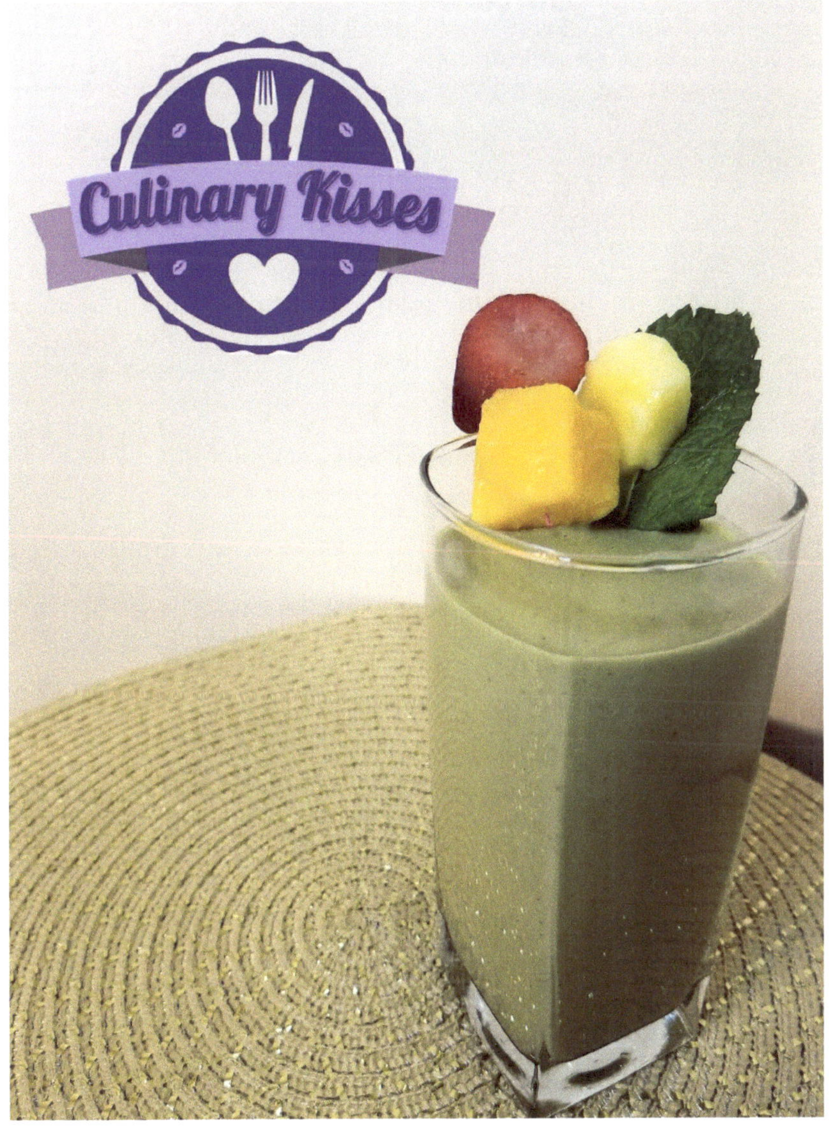

NUTRITIONAL INFO

Kale is one of the most nutrient-dense foods on the planet with an amazingly high content of vitamin A, C, and K per cup (206%, 134%, and 684% respectively). It's a cruciferous vegetable that's a member of the cabbage family.

Kale is also loaded with powerful antioxidants and can help lower cholesterol; which will also reduce the risk of heart disease.

Spinach is a super green leafy vegetable ranks high in vitamin A, potassium, magnesium, calcium, folate (vitamin B9), and iron. It's important to get iron from your diet, because the amount of iron in the body determines how efficiently the body uses energy. Just be sure to combine it with citrus fruits to improve absorption. Spinach also contains an antioxidant that has been shown to lower glucose levels, increase insulin sensitivity, and possibly help people with diabetes.

Cinnamon is a spice that's native to South American, Southeast Asia, and the Caribbean. In ancient times, cinnamon was used to treat chronic coughing, arthritis, and sore throats. It's also known to be good for treating digestive problems and diabetes. Cinnamon is also high in calcium, packing in 26mg per teaspoon, and in potassium with 11mg.

Strawberries are so amazing that they allow their seeds to grow on the outside, versus the inside, of the fruit. One normal size berry packs in 18mg of potassium. They're also an excellent source of vitamin C, manganese, and antioxidants. These antioxidants may have benefits for heart health and blood sugar control. Strawberries are also 91% water and score low on the glycemic index (which means they're considered safe for people with diabetes).

Nutmeg is a spice that is typically used sparingly. It has been known to treat insomnia, help with digestion, combat bad breath, relieve pain, and improve blood circulation.
Nutmeg also has a calming effect when ingested in small amounts.

Mangoes, like strawberries, are an excellent source for antioxidants. They're low in calories and high in vitamins A, C, and E. Vitamin C is one of the most important antioxidants; as it's necessary for the formation of collagen (the protein that provides the skin's elasticity).

Mangoes are also rich in iron and folate, but don't peel them because the skin may have antioxidant and anti-inflammatory properties.

Blueberries are considered to be the King of antioxidants! One cup of these bluish-purple berries contain 35% vitamin K, 25% manganese, and 24% vitamin C. Not only are they tasty (sweet) and convenient (small, portable), but blueberries are also low in calories and high in nutrients. As a matter of fact, they're some of the most nutrient-dense berries. They've been deemed a superfood and rightfully so. And as if that wasn't enough, blueberries have also been known to lower blood pressure.

Pumpkin seeds (AKA Pepitas) are high in antioxidants, magnesium, and fiber. They're considered nutritional powerhouses because:
- (a) They're a great source of magnesium, iron, B vitamins, and protein
- (b) They're known to have anti-inflammatory properties

Pumpkin seeds have also been linked to lowering blood sugar levels, improving prostate and bladder health, and reducing the risk of certain cancers.

Pineapple may contain disease-fighting antioxidants, reduce the risk of cancer, boost immunity, and suppress inflammation. They may reduce the recovery time after surgery or strenuous exercise. Pineapples enzymes can potentially aid in digestion and in combating belly fat.

Coconut is a healthy fat and has been known to help raise the levels of HDL, or the good cholesterol. As if that wasn't good enough, coconuts are also rich in vitamin B6, magnesium, zinc, manganese, and selenium. Coconuts are also high in iron and copper, which help form red blood cells.

Interesting fact, coconut is classified as a "grass."

Allspice is a berry, even though the name alludes to it being a spice. It's an unripe, dried berry from the Pimento tree. The English renamed it allspice because it has hints of pepper, cloves, cinnamon, nutmeg, and juniper. Allspice has many "anti" health benefits including anti-inflammatory, antioxidant, antiseptic, antiviral, and antifungal. It's also been known to help fight cancer.

Walnuts are known as a super source of omega-3s. They may also decrease inflammation, promote a healthy gut, support weight control, lower blood pressure, manage type 2 diabetes, and reduce the risk of some cancers. Sounds like walnuts have earned their superfood status.

THE CULINARY KISSES 5-DAY DETOX: A MADE-EASY MEAL PLAN

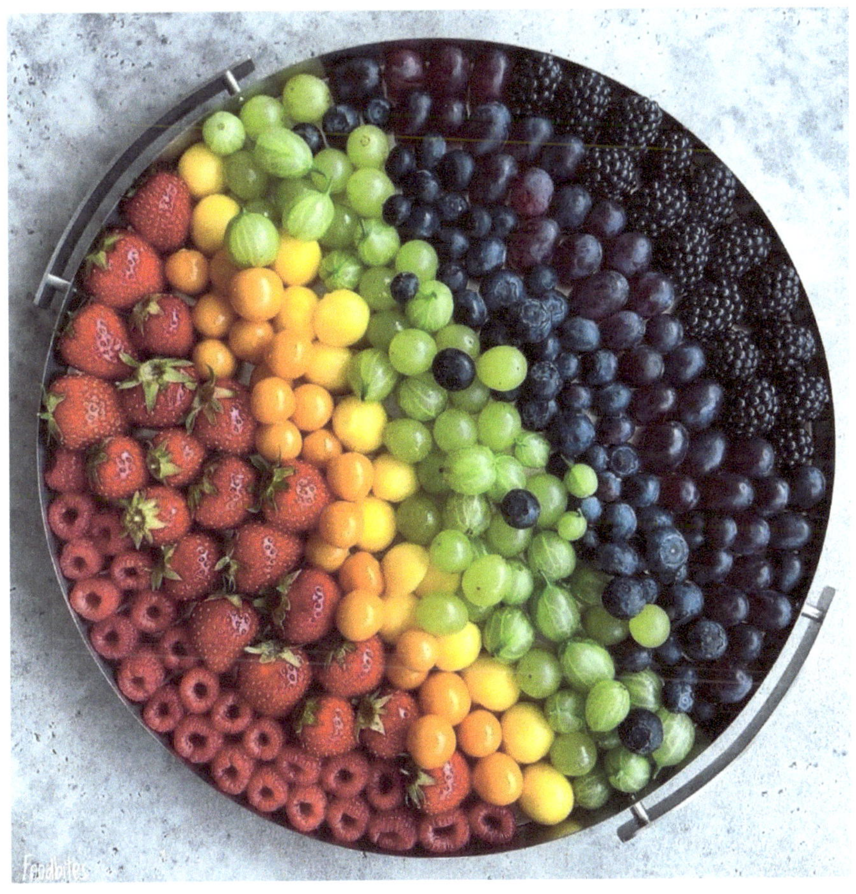

EAT THE RAINBOW

DETOX SNACKS

Smoothies are meant to start your day off right, to break your fast when you wake up, and to pump your body full of vitamins and nutrients. Snacks, however, are used to supplement your diet in between meals. This is why healthy snack options are important. They should follow the 5-DAY DETOX Guidelines the same as your smoothies and your meals.
Some tasty yet nutrient-dense options of snacks during the detox include:

*Fresh fruit
*Detox or herbal tea with raw almonds
*Pears and blueberries
*Spa water
*An apple with raw walnuts
*A mini snack plate that includes raw nuts and seeds with a
  variety of fresh fruit

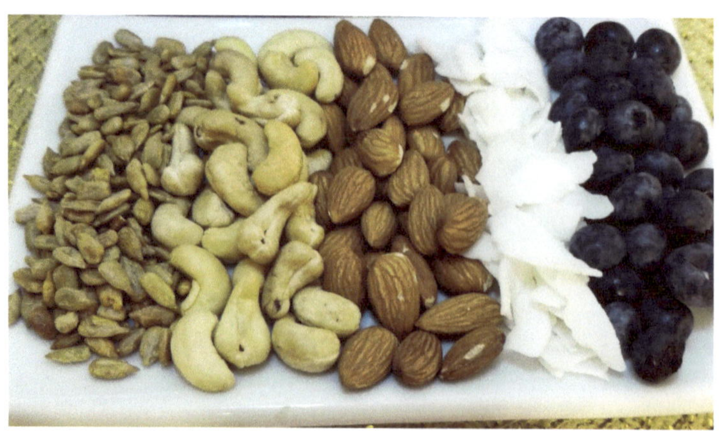

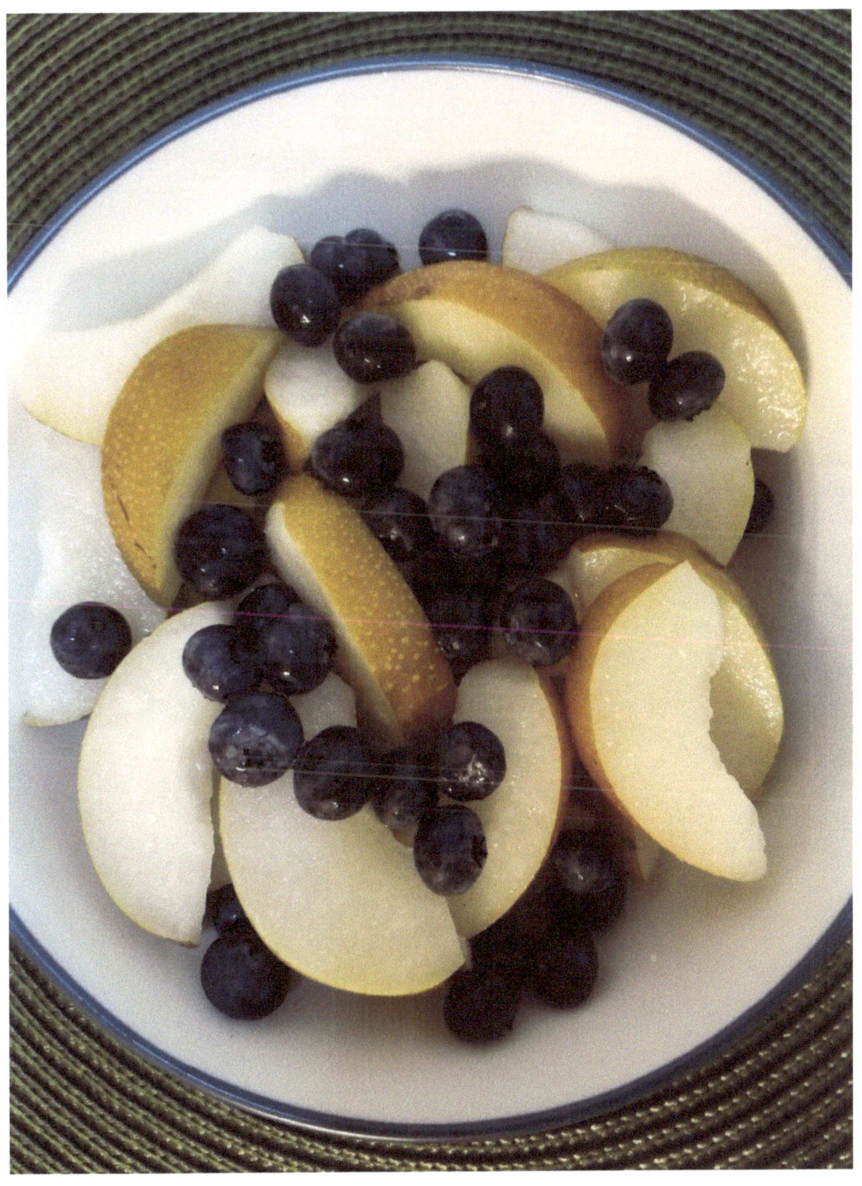

<u>DETOX MEALS</u>

Detox Meals consist of a collage of nutritious, colorful small plates. A little bit of this with a little bit of that will do the trick. Think plant-based "meatless" Mondays or what I like to call "mix and match meals." That's when you take something that's already cooked in your refrigerator and cook something to go along with it to create a full meal. Let's say, for example, you have some green beans and butternut squash already done, and you cook some quinoa and red beans to go with them. That's a "mix and match meal." Here are some ideas of how you can put together creative yet delicious Detox Meals …

GRAINS
Amaranth
Barley
Brown rice
Bulgur
Farro
Freekeh
Kamut
Millet
Oats
Teff
Wild rice

GREENS
Arugula
Collards
Dandelions
Kale
Mustards
Rapini
Romaine
Spinach
Swiss chard

OTHER
Brussel sprouts
Cabbage
Squash

BEANS
Adzuki
Black
Butter
Cannellini
Cranberry
Garbanzo
Great northern
Kidney
Lentils
Lima
Navy
Pinto
Red
Split pea

ROOTS
Beets
Carrots
Fennel
Garlic
Ginger
Onions
Radish
Rutabaga
Sweet potatoes
Turmeric
Turnips

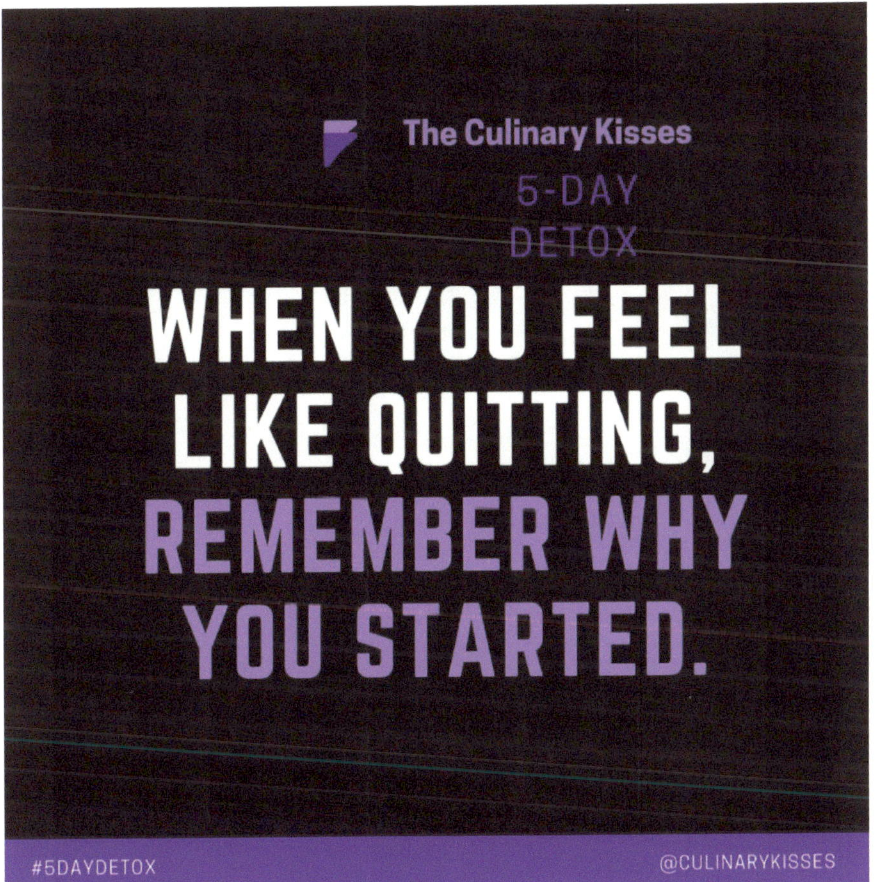
The Culinary Kisses
5-DAY
DETOX
WHEN YOU FEEL
LIKE QUITTING,
REMEMBER WHY
YOU STARTED.
#5DAYDETOX
@CULINARYKISSES

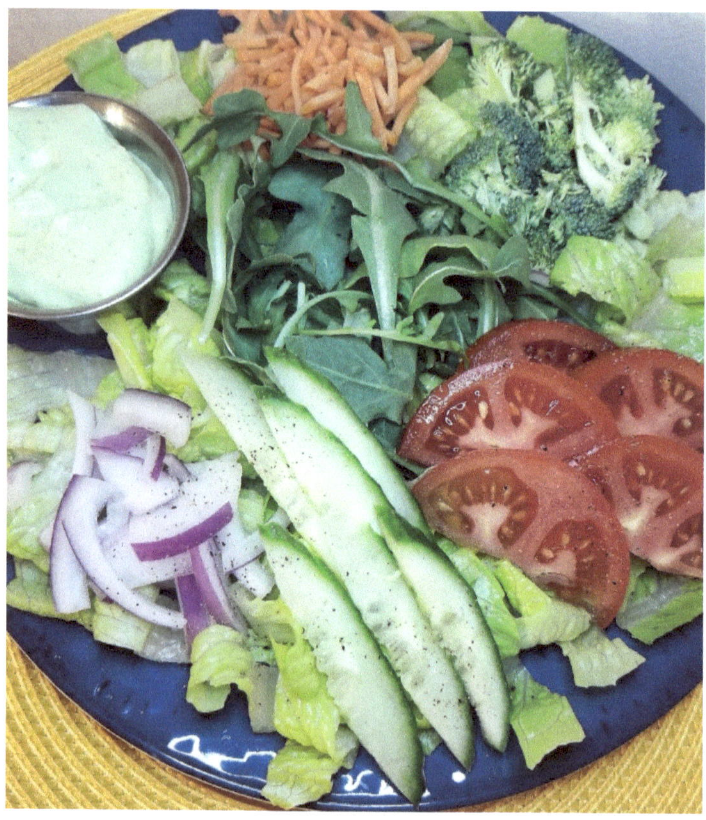

Subscribe to our blog "From the Catwalk to the Kitchen" for our Detox recipes and subscribe to our You Tube channel for instructional videos on how to create delicious "mix and match meals!"

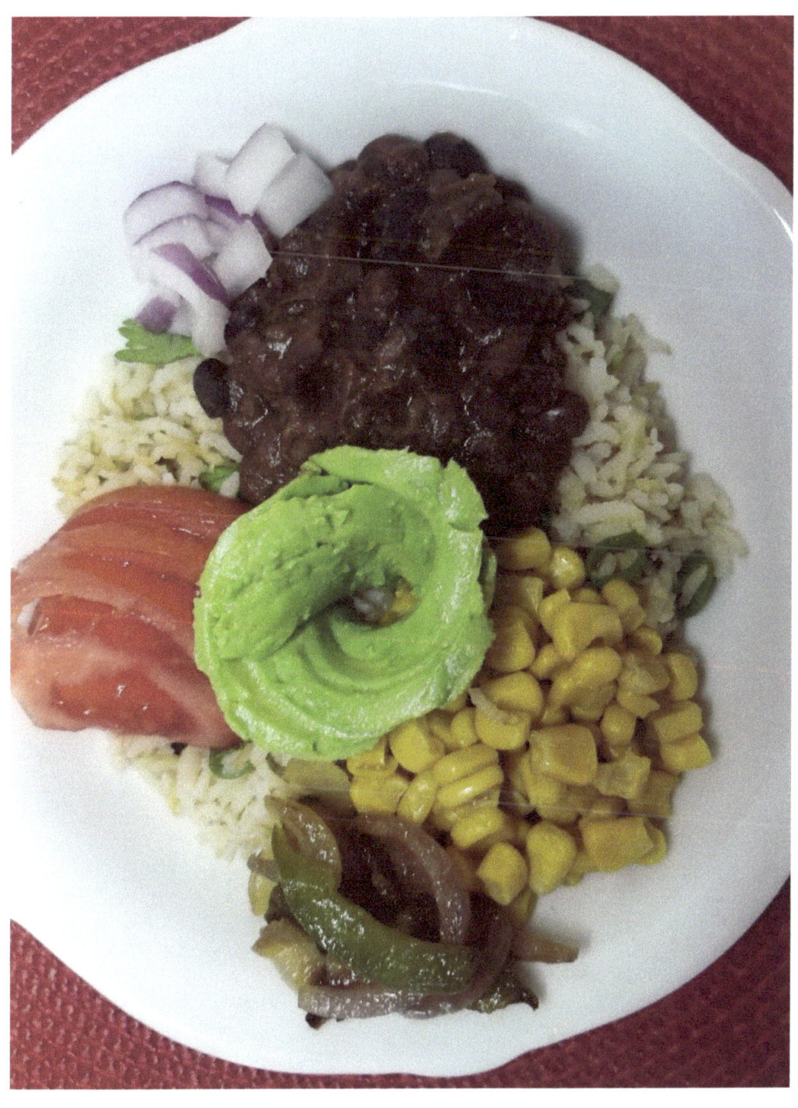

<u>DETOX DESSERTS</u>

You may think having dessert is totally out of the question when you're detoxing, but that's not necessarily true. There are foods, or food combinations, that will curb your sweet cravings.
Of course there's fruit … strawberries, blueberries, grapes, apples, etc. Yes, but there's more. Why not cut some apples into chunks, place them in a covered pot on medium low heat, and let them cook low for about 40 minutes. Then sprinkle with ground cinnamon, add a dash of ground nutmeg, a drop of vanilla, and then stir. Voila, you have homemade apple sauce!

Another alternative, although it's high in (healthy) fat, is to make chia seed pudding with a fresh fruit reduction. It's especially nice when topped with some almond slivers for crunch.

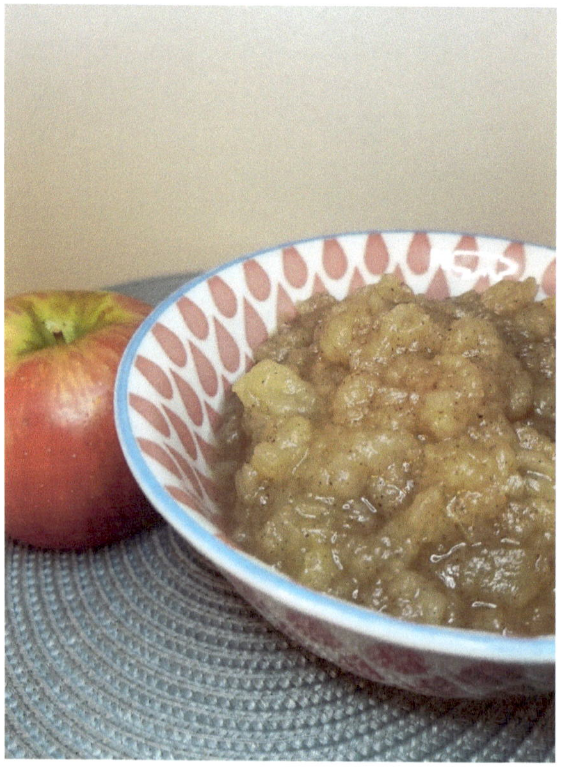

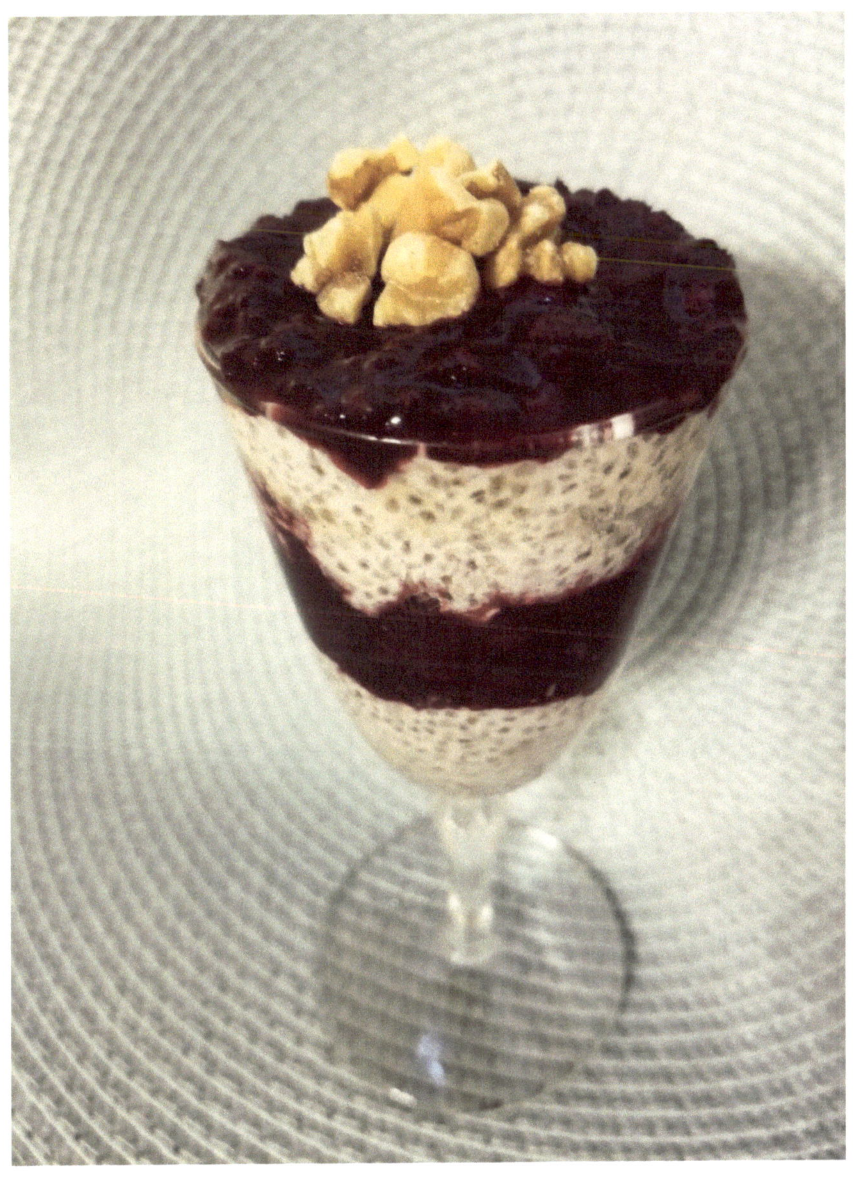

THE CULINARY KISSES 5-DAY DETOX PROGRAM

That's it! It's just that simple. No counting calories or points, and no measuring meals or waistlines. Remember, you're eating to maximize nutrients, to feed your cells, and to cleanse your body. Following these detox guidelines (along with incorporating at least 20 minutes of cardio exercise a few times a week) will improve your health AND your self-esteem.

Good luck on your detox journey.

Wishing you continual health and happiness …

Food & Kisses,
Chef Angela-Michelle

Watch a video on how to make the detox smoothies →
https://youtu.be/MDLo-YyA4r0

Follow Culinary Kisses on all Social Media outlets using @culinarykisses

Check out the website at www.CulinaryKisses.com

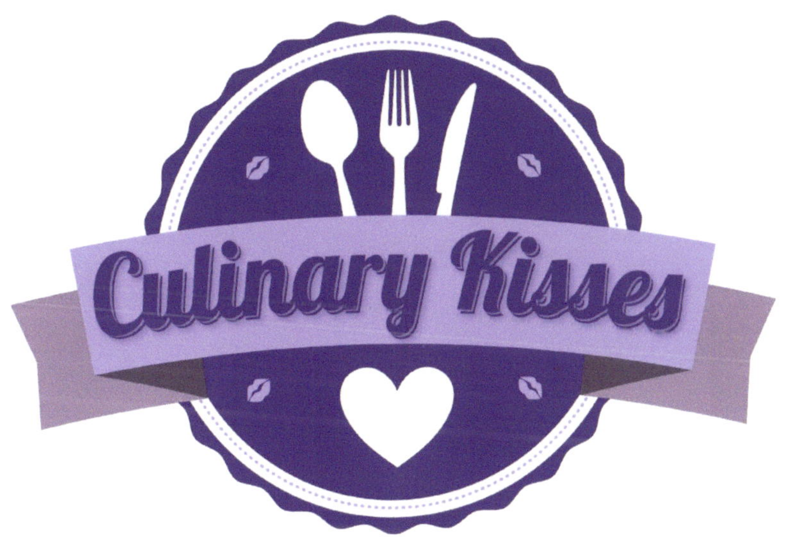

www.CulinaryKisses.com

www.ingramcontent.com/pod-product-compliance
Lightning Source LLC
Chambersburg PA
CBHW040251240726
48664CB00001B/356